Terms and Conditions

LEGAL NOTICE

Table Of Contents

Foreword

Of the many things that we do just instinctively and do not give much of a thought to, sleep is probably the most prominent one. Most of us sleep only because we have to. We sleep because we cannot stay awake all 24 hours in the day.

Instead of sleep being something that we need to keep our bodies charged and maintain our health and wellbeing, most of us regard it as an obligation... something that nature has ordained us to do and hence we have to follow it.

However, this is definitely not the view held by the several health experts, meditation gurus, spiritual gurus and sleep counselors. According to these people, one should not sleep out of compulsion. Just like how we plan what to eat and spend a significant part of the day in planning and preparing our meals, sleep needs to be planned as well. It is not enough just to have a nice bedroom with a cozy bed to sleep in.

Sleep patterning is a concept that is becoming quite popular in recent times. Health experts tell people that they have to maintain regular sleep patterns if they want to ensure that their health is in top condition. This is not done as easily as one thinks. Planning is needed.

It is also important to make sleep a part of our lifestyle. Or, to put it better, we should create a lifestyle in which sleep is given its due prominence. It is only when we are able to do that that we can unleash the tremendous healing effects of sleep. Yes, sleep does have

healing benefits, and, as most people think, these healing benefits aren't just confined to our psychological state; they also pour out into our physical being. Good sleep is needed for our mental as well as physical enhancement.

In this eBook, *Sleep Sanctuary—Salvation for the Sleep-Deprived*, I am going to deal with three important aspects. I am not going to divide these three aspects into different sections, because that would not be the right way to do so, but I am going to intersperse them everywhere throughout this e-Book.

These three aspects are:-

→ *Why is sleep important to our wellbeing?* This will be followed by several discussions on why we just cannot do without the right amount of sleep in our lives.

→ *Why do some people have sleep problems and why these problems are becoming more acute in recent times?* Here we shall talk about problems such as sleep apnea, insomnia, restlessness and other problems that keep us away from getting adequate amounts of sleeps. The focus will be on present times, because today we are sleeping less than ever before. This is bringing in its wake a host of problems, and one of the reasons why we are visiting a lot more doctors today than before is because we do not sleep well.

→ *What can we do to improve our sleep patterns?* This is the most important part of the eBook and you will find the information strewn throughout. With several illustrations, tips and strategies, I shall endeavor to tell you what we can do to

improve our sleep patterns, especially in today's sleep-deprived times.

I would ironically request you to "wake up" and read this eBook on sleep deprivation! That's because you have to pay full attention to this; it is something that will tell you what's missing in your life, and why. Wake up, smell the coffee, and plan to live a lifestyle in which sleep gets its due importance.

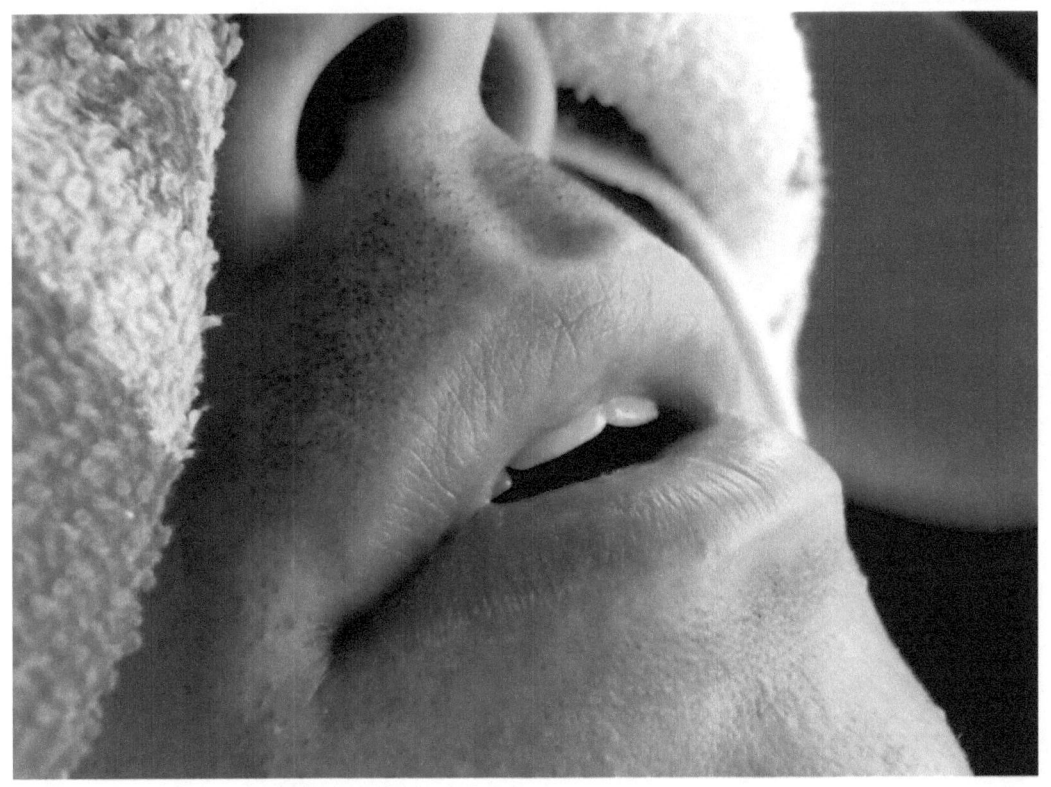

Sleeping Sanctuary - Salvation For The Sleep Deprived

The Ultimate Guide To Sleeping, Napping, Resting And Restoring Your Energy

Chapter 1:

What's So Good about Sleep Anyway?

Synopsis

At the outset, it is best to understand why sleep is so important to us, especially in today's day and age. Our general health has degenerated in recent times; that's a fact no one can detract. Now, there are several reasons why our health has taken a tumble. We are moving away from nature and our own natural body patterns each day that we live. Our food has become synthetic for its most part, the clothes that we wear and most of the things that we use are not natural at all, even our civilization itself is completely away from the rule book of nature.

It is for this reason that we are facing so many health perils today. And, one of the most profound elements that is sordidly missing from our lifestyle is a healthy sleep pattern.

In this chapter, we shall see why sleep is important. Why is it important for us to devote at least 7 to 9 hours of our day to sleep? How does sleeplessness or sleep deprivation affect our lives? These are important questions to answer before we move along with things.

What's So Good about Sleep Anyway?

Finding time to sleep in our busy schedules is extremely important for our health and wellbeing. Most people push the boundaries when it comes to sleep. We restrict the time we allow for sleep, going to bed progressively later as we try to fit in the many different jobs that need completion each day. We underestimate the importance of sleep. Without adequate sleep our bodies will react, and those important schedules we put off sleep to achieve, will be affected eventually.

It's only recently that we have begun to fully understand just how much our body needs sleep to function properly. Most of the body's normal activities rely on us having a regular sleep and an interrupted sleep pattern is a significant stress on our bodies.

Our nervous system, our digestive system and the ability of our body to repair itself are all dependent on our sleep cycles being consistent and regular. When we deprive our body of sleep, we inhibit our brains ability to make decision, our emotional responses to situations may be compromised, and even how we interact socially may be affected.

Sleep is as necessary for our health as eating and drinking is. It has long been recognized that sleep deprivation is an effective torture tool, and experiments using rats have revealed that they their live expectancy is significantly reduced when they are sleep deprived under experimental conditions.

How much sleep a person needs is dependent on factors such as age and gender. Pregnant women for example, may require more sleep than a non-pregnant woman of the same age group and a child may require more sleep than an adult, however an older adult generally requires less sleep than a younger adult.

The amount of sleep an individual needs is fairly consistent with their age group. A typical adult will require approximately 7-9 hours of sleep a night to maintain optimum health and performance. If we reduce that amount of sleep time over a series of nights, our body will eventually react and we need to make up that time, usually in what is termed as a "sleep in".

However, even though we know we will sleep in on the weekend, our performance during the working week may be severely affected by our lack of sleep. If we find ourselves excessively yawning during the day, or finding it difficult to remember simple details or make simple judgment calls correctly, it is possible we are suffering from sleep deprivation.

People take micro sleeps where they lose consciousness for very short periods of time without realizing it, leading to potentially dangerous situations. Many road deaths and incidents at work have been directly traced to insufficient sleep the night before. With so many serious side effects and consequences of not sleeping, we should all be ensuring we schedule adequate sleep into our daily lives.

Chapter 2:

But I Am Not Tired... I Won't Sleep!

Synopsis

A very important aspect of sleep deprivation that the world is facing today, and probably a contributor to that as well, is our own unwillingness to sleep. We know that sleep is important; we even know that if we do not sleep adequately, then it will create a lot of problems for us in future, but we are still in denial and we do not give this very essential part of our lives its due importance.

What is it that is making us *not sleep*? There are so many people who are burning the midnight lamp for various reasons, but to what avail? Are deadlines so important that we should lose sleep over them? What effects can such a hazardous lifestyle have on our health?

In this chapter, we are going to see what makes people lose sleep. We learn, through the concept of Circadian Rhythms, that our body is made to behave in a particular way. The mechanism of our body ordains that it should sleep, and the amount of sleep it gets should be adequate.

But I Am Not Tired... I Won't Sleep!

We all know if we are "morning" people or "evening" people. Many people can jump out of bed easily in the morning, often without the need for an alarm clock. At 9 pm in the evening they are ready to sleep, their ability to focus and think clearly severely diminished. Yet they may be married to someone who finds it extremely difficult to get out of bed in the mornings, but at 9 pm at night they are awake and produce their best quality work.

The difference between this pair is their biological clock that affects what are called the Circadian Rhythms. The hormone melatonin, which is produced in the brain in response to darkness, increases at night and is decreased during the day. Melatonin makes you feel drowsy and reduces your body temperature. Blood levels of the hormone are highest around midnight and levels gradually reduce in the second half of the night.

Every individual has his or her own minor variation to this hormonal response. This variation is the reason why some people feel sleepy earlier than others. Age is also a contributing factor to our sleep needs.

The area that controls the production of melatonin also controls other body functions such as blood pressure and urine production which are reduced at night.

The wake sleep cycle is the rise and fall of melatonin and the response of our body to its production or lack of production are the symptoms we feel when we are tired and the alert feelings we have when we are

awake during periods when there are low levels of melatonin circulating in our blood.

The levels of melatonin reducing once you are exposed to day light explains why you gradually feel more energetic and less sleepy after you have been awake for a while.

Many people believe that their morning coffee is essential for them to wake up, but while to a degree this is true as caffeine is a stimulant, simultaneously your body's levels of melatonin are reducing under the influence of the day light creating a more alert feeling and less drowsiness which is stimulated further by your cup of coffee or tea.

The amount of sleep we need and the reason why we don't always feel sleepy at night, and yet feel very sleepy in the afternoon after a big meal, or on a hot day is dependent on a number of factors. There are other reasons for feeling less than energetic in the afternoon, which must be addressed.

The types of food we eat for lunch for example will affect our afternoon energy levels, but some people do experience a slight rise in melatonin levels in the afternoon and a slight drop in body temperature, and while this does not have the same effect as night time melatonin, it does cause drowsiness and a need for daytime naps.

Chapter 3:

Does Counting Sheep Really Work?

Synopsis

A lot of people around us, people walking the face of the earth just as we do, are deprived. They are deprived of sleep. Sleep is a natural gift, but these people have taken their lives so far away from the rule of nature that they have quite literally lost sleep.

However, sleep is something that we just cannot do without, isn't it? Even if people have been walking on the wild side where sleep is concerned, a time comes when they try to call it back. They want a healthy sleeping pattern to be formulated in their lives once again, and most of these people are prepared to do several logical and illogical things for it.

People try everything from meditation to medication; they try to improve their breathing patterns, they try to imbibe new relaxation methods within themselves... all this is an unending quest to call sleep back into their nocturnal, and sometimes even diurnal, lives.

But, do these methods work? Can lost sleep be regained? This chapter delves into such methods and reveals which of these sleep-inducing methods work and which do not.

And, yes, also keep your eyes out to read about whether old wives' tales like counting sheep work if you are looking for good sleep.

Does Counting Sheep Really Work?

Have you ever tried counting sheep in the hope it will help you sleep? When you are feeling tired but you can't sleep, it can be very frustrating. Approximately half of all people in the USA experience trouble sleeping. In desperation, many of them try medications, meditations; in fact, anything they can think of, to help them relax and sleep. Do these techniques work and end the insomnia (inability to sleep)?

Counting sheep sounds like "an old wives tale". It can work, and psychologists have shown that it probably works by focusing both sides of your brain on the one subject, not giving you chance to think about other things that keep your brain active.

Other people try medications. Most are supplied on prescription with medical supervisions. There are two main types of "sleeping" tablets; the tablets to help you fall asleep and others that will help you to stay asleep. Many people do notice an immediate improvement in their sleeping patterns when they take medications, however the body quickly develops a tolerance to them and they have a rebound effect that has the opposite reaction to their intended use. In other words, if you take sleeping tablets over a long period of time, it is probable you will start to have insomnia problems even though you are taking the medications.

There are many remedies popular with insomniacs and all have their supporters who will tell you they work. These include having a hot drink or bath before bed, not drinking caffeinated drinks after a certain time of day and restricting stimulating activities, like exercise before bed. Each of these remedies have their rationale rooted in the idea of allowing your body time to relax and prepare itself for sleep and reducing activities that include the use of light, which prevents the release of melatonin.

For most people, preparing the bedroom and yourself for sleep can help promote sleep and there is plenty of research suggesting that everyone, even those who don't suffer from insomnia should allow time to prepare for bed and to keep the bedroom for activities that contribute to sleep and don't stimulate the brain. Using favorite relaxation techniques before bed such as prayer or yoga or meditation may help you feel ready for bed. Ensuring the room is dark, there are no illuminated clocks or computers that create light, may also create optimum conditions for sleep.

It is important to remember that insomnia though it affects so many people and interferes with many normal body functions, anxiety over the condition is likely to create stress and tension and increase the chances of insomnia continuing. If you are not able to sleep, especially if it is not a regular problem for you, don't lie in bed but worrying about it, but try to use some of the relaxation techniques mentioned. Seek medical attention if the insomnia continues.

Chapter 4:

I Need More Sleep... I Never Seem to Have Had Enough

Synopsis

Sleep deprivation means that we do not get the sleep that we need for our proper wellbeing. This is a precarious road that all of us are treading currently. We are compromising with our sleep for various reasons. The human body needs to sleep for 7 to 9 hours each day, but hardly are we getting that. One of the biggest problems lies in our faulty scheduling of our time. We are not able to manage things effectively and that is why we end up spending our sleep time doing other things, like that work we bring home from the office.

This is definitely dangerous territory. If we are not able to sleep effectively, then we spend the next day getting tired and restless. We aren't able to put in our creative best. Our thought patterns begin to falter. Our mind gets clouded with various psychological problems and the difficulties begin to crop up.

That is where this feeling starts cropping in. We sleep, but we do not find it to be adequate. Something somewhere, something vital, seems to be missing. We want to put in more hours of rest, but it doesn't happen.

Health experts are also talking right now about the so-called 'sleep debt' a concept that should scare most people who are living a rapid lifestyle today. This sleep debt is about how our lost sleep will one day catch up with us. Nature has decreed that we should spend one-third of our life sleeping. If we do not do that, then it can imperil us in some way. A lot of people feel that they can keep up through the night just on cups of coffee, but it doesn't work that way. We may be pushing sleep back as much as we can, but we must also know that this lost sleep will manifest itself in the form of health problems at some time or the other.

Sleep deprivation is the reason we feel tired all the time, why we are not able to put in our best.

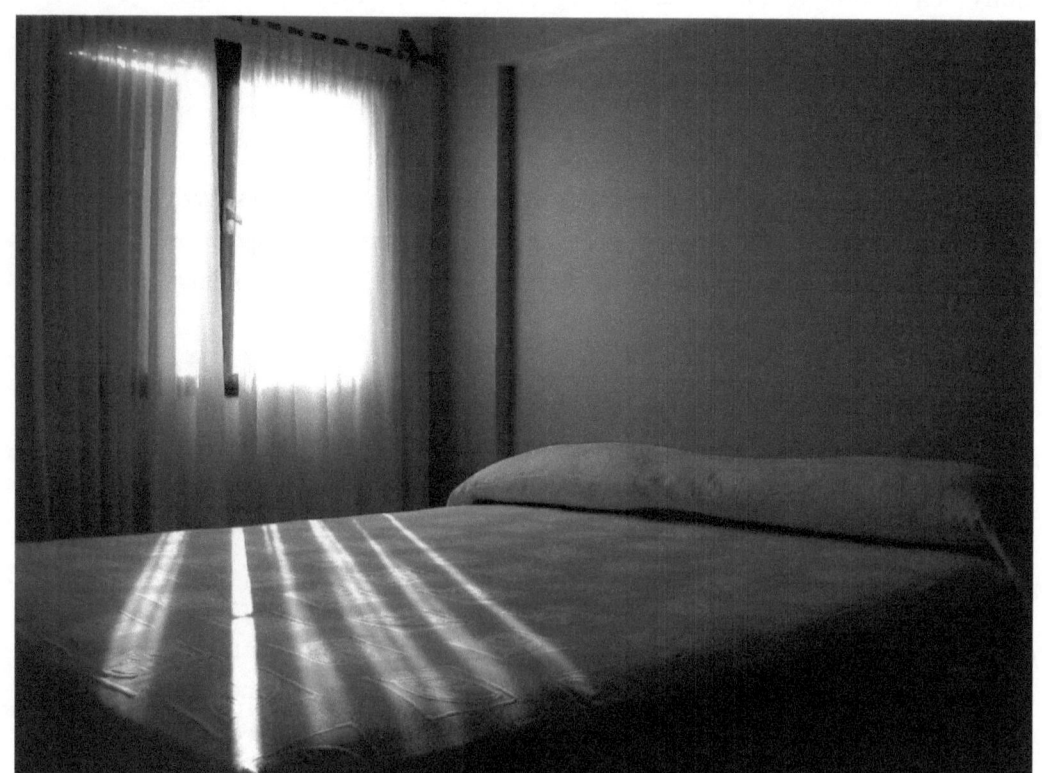

I Need More Sleep... I Never Seem to Have Had Enough

Are you one of those people who have a normal night's sleep (7-9 hours), yet you still feel tired during the day? Have you ever wondered why you just cannot seem to go for more than a few hours without feeling you need a sleep?

During the evening, conditions work together to create optimum conditions for the release of melatonin, a hormone that is released into our blood streams and produce the drowsiness that alerts us to "feeling tired" and ready for bed at night. Some people experience a release of this hormone in the afternoon and it is responsible for the feeling of lethargy and tiredness in the early afternoon.

There are many people however, who experience this drowsiness for other reasons. Certain medical conditions can affect people, which even though they may have a regular sleep and waking pattern and spend the average number of hours in bed sleeping, they are still not receiving adequate sleep for their body to function without drowsiness during the day.

Some of the most common of these disorders include:-

Sleep Apnea

If you snore when you sleep, it is highly likely you may also have a condition known as sleep apnea. People with this condition actually stop breathing for short periods while they are sleeping. This causes a drop in blood oxygen levels, and the brain disturbs the sleep of the person to ensure they breathe. If this happens regularly through the night, it will make you tired throughout the day.

Limb Movements

Some people are affected at night by the need to move their legs and limbs due to "restless legs" a syndrome that causes tingling or other unusual sensations in the limbs. Other people experience sudden movements in their limbs and this causes their legs or arms to jerk suddenly and without warning. Both of these conditions, even if they occur subconsciously will interfere with the sleep cycle and disturb sleep.

Medical Reasons

There are large groups of people who fall asleep during the day for very short periods of time regularly. These micro-sleeps maybe hereditary or maybe caused by some brain dysfunction.

If you or a loved one experience any of these symptoms and feel tired and often feel tired throughout the day you should seek medical advice.

Feeling tired throughout the day may also be simply a result of the food we eat during the day. Research is showing that foods that are highly processed and high in carbohydrates may raise our blood sugar levels suddenly and create a sudden drop in the afternoon creating the afternoon lethargy most of us know very well. Having a lunch that includes protein and ensuring that exercise is included in the days routine may help to reverse the effect of this very common reason for feeling sleepy during the day despite a good night's sleep.

Chapter 5:

An Hour before Midnight Is Worth Two after

Synopsis

In this chapter, we shall be answering some vital questions about sleep. We know that we all need to sleep adequately, but how much is really enough? In this chapter, we will speak about how many hours of sleep do we need really.

Also, the hours that we sleep are important. It matters at what time we go to sleep and at what time we wake up. Our wellbeing depends not only on the duration of our sleep, but it also depends on the exact timings of our sleep.

We shall be seeing the best time to sleep in this chapter.

In the process, we shall be putting to rest some old wives' tales about sleep. What is real and what is just a superstition? Read on to know more about sleep.

An Hour before Midnight Is Worth Two after

Most of us remember going to bed early as young children and our bedtime getting progressively later as we progressed into our teen years. As adults, we probably have an idea on the amount of sleep we generally need to feel in optimum condition the following day. We know the effect that a late night will have, especially if it is followed by an early morning and a long day at work.

Most adults require 7-9 hours of sleep a night, although for others it is very individual with many requiring a greater or less need. Young babies under 3 months old, tend to have high levels of melatonin in their circulation and sleep long hours under its influence.

As their pineal gland matures, the biological clock starts to develop regular wake and sleep cycles and babies and young children gradually need less hours of sleep. Young children will still require approximately 10 hours sleep at night and adolescents may require 9- 10 hours a night.

As adults age, they will wake more regularly at night either due to health related reasons or because they are sleeping lighter and their sleep is more often interrupted. Older people often need to sleep during the day to compensate for the disturbed sleep patterns at night With the busy lifestyles, we lead and the attraction of home entertainment and computers, many people are sleep deprived. They go to bed too late and wake up too early and eventually the body will respond physically to this lack of sleep.

Researchers suggest that sleeping before midnight may have significant health benefits particularly to body functions and cardiac health. Research continues to determine if the important factor in the relationship between health and sleep is how many hours a person actually sleeps, or when they actually sleep and if an early bedtime offers health advantages over a later one.

What is definitely emerging in all studies is the reduction in blood pressure readings and decreased circulating fats in those who have the recommended number of hours of sleep at night. Those who sleep before midnight appeared to have less physical symptoms of cardiac disorders than those who slept after midnight.

Most experts speculate that the later we go to sleep, the greater the potential of interfering with our biological clock. This has the potential for the development of significant health problems. Maybe as a child, you used to talk of going to bed early being a means of staying smart, making money and having fewer health problems, and the evidence is definitely supporting this famous children's rhyme.

The research certainly indicates that people who become disciplined with a more scheduled approach to the time they wake and the time they sleep will have immediate and long-term health benefits. This resets the body clock and reduces the incidence of insomnia.

Chapter 6:

6 Tips for a Power Nap

Synopsis

Our current lifestyle is such that we may not get adequate sleep during the night. We often need to keep up late hours because we have so much work to do or because we are socializing, and that can be a problem for our sleep timings. To add to that, we might also need to wake up early in the morning, which could wreck our schedule too.

That is the reason why some people have invented the idea of a power nap. A power nap is a short nap, usually of just a few hours, during which you sleep in a sound and undisturbed manner, and wake up feeling totally refreshed. Hitherto considered impossible, now more and more people are trying out power naps and are succeeding at them too. They are finding that taking such short power naps throughout the day keeps them perked up and they can do more than they usually do with their deprived sleep routines.

Power naps have several physiological benefits as well. They are not just about giving us some much-needed sleep, but they can actually help us biologically. We may live longer because of power naps. We are going to see about these benefits as well.

6 Tips for a Power Nap

Most people are more than aware of how difficult it can be to stay awake in the heat of the middle parts of the day. As the early afternoon approaches, many of us find it difficult to stay awake. We become drowsy and find it very difficult to focus and complete our work. Some people find they hallucinate or fall asleep for a few minutes. These situations can be extremely dangerous, especially if handling electrical equipment or driving a car.

Why we feel that sleepy is due to many factors. Our internal body clock and our natural body rhythms, the temperature of the environment we are working in, the lighting in that environment, how much time we spend working on computers and what we eat for our breaks all play an important role on how we feel in the afternoon.

There is growing evidence that a 20-minute nap in the afternoon improves focus and memory, which increases productivity and workplace safety. Those who work at home or who are in a position to take this "power" nap, will benefit from it and should take advantage of the opportunity to have one whenever they can.

Many cultures around the world have recognized the need to close shops, schools, and businesses and include an afternoon siesta into the daily routine. Today, in the fast-paced lifestyles of the industrialized world are embracing the afternoon nap, not so much as a luxury, but a necessity to help them deal with the many expectations on their time in the afternoon and evening.

Workplaces around the world are providing space for their staff to take a power nap, recognizing the benefit to the workplace when staff

does have time to take one. If this is not possible in your workplace, there are things you can do:-

→ Take a 10-minute nap in your car or in another safe area during your lunch break. Even these ten minutes could mean a lot to you. However, when you are preparing yourself to take such a short nap, make sure to free your mind of all distractions just surrender yourself completely to sleep. Maybe you could use some soothing music to help you free your mind completely. When you wake up, you will feel the difference.

→ Take some time during your lunch break to include exercise. Physical exercise improves circulation of the blood, improves oxygen levels in the blood, and raises body temperature all of which reduces drowsiness and fatigue. Consequently, when you try to take a power nap later in the day, you will find that the short surrender to sleep comes more easily to you. If you keep working your body effectively, then sleep patterns will definitely improve and you will find the difference in these short power naps you take as well.

→ Eat lunch that is not high in sugar or carbohydrates. Include protein sources such as low fat cheese, meat or chicken to reduce the chance of a sudden drop in blood sugar levels which create a lack of energy and feelings of drowsiness. Heavy foods have a tendency to make you lose sleep, and even if you do fall asleep, your sleep will be highly erratic. The best way is to keep a light meal, which helps you psychologically as well.

→ Go for a walk and increase the amount of natural light in your work area to reduce melatonin production levels in the afternoon. Apart from that, the walk in natural beauty that you take will also help your body to control its mind in a better way and, resultantly, you will be able to sleep better.

→ Join a meditation class, especially Yoga. In these classes, you will be taught how you can control your mind. This is a very important thing to learn, especially in today's times. When you learn how to control your mind, you will be able to switch it 'on' or 'off' as desired. This can go a long way in improving your health. Firstly, you will be taught through various *asanas*, mainly the *Shavasana*, that you can completely surrender your body and let it loose in both the physiological and psychological sense. This helps us to free ourselves from our bodies for a while, and the body goes to sleep. This is a wonderful way to find those important snatches of sleep, wherever you are. You may not be able to perform the *Shavasana* at all times, but you will certainly be able to learn how to have those all-important power naps whenever you need to.

→ You can have a short power nap in your swiveling chair itself. All you have to do is to lock the door and tell people not to disturb you for the next 20 minutes. Then, pull the shades if you can, settle in the most comfortable position you can on the chair and close your eyes. Free your mind from all its thoughts, or think about something pleasant. You will find that sleep encompasses you soon, and you will have your power nap.

When you have these power naps, in the beginning you may find it difficult to wake up at the right time. But as time passes, this will become a habit. Initially, you may have to set an alarm on your cell phone to wake you up or you may have to tell someone to do that. However, soon your body's system will adjust to the new routine and you will find out that you are able to sleep more easily, and wake up on dot.

These simple steps may help reduce the afternoon drowsiness and enable you to function in the afternoons with as much productivity as when you arrived at work that morning. Combining them with a regular time to wake up and go to bed and a healthy lifestyle approach to diet and exercise will help you feel more energized and able to increase your personal productivity.

Binaural Beats

When we are having a discussion on power naps, it is relevant to speak about binaural beats as well. Binaural beats are a specific kind of music, which are made up of specific natural sounds that have a soothing effect on the human body. You might find sounds like birds chirping, insects humming, grass swishing in the breeze, ocean waves moving in rhythm and such others in these binaural beats.

When you are preparing for your power nap, just play this music. You will experience the benefits right away. You will find that, as soon as the music begins to play, your mind will surrender itself to the rhythm of the beats. As these are mostly natural sounds, your mind will completely give itself up to them.

A typical binaural beats track lasts around 20 minutes. This is exactly the time you require for your power nap. You could get this kind of music in MP3 form, downloadable from the Internet. Get it on your MP3 player or iPod and use it whenever you want. Just shut your eyes and let the music play. You will soon fall asleep, and you will see a vast difference when you wake up.

Even if you are suffering from problems such as sleeplessness (insomnia), binaural beats can help. A lot of people are recommended using this music at night so that they can get proper sleep, and not have to toss and turn in bed for long.

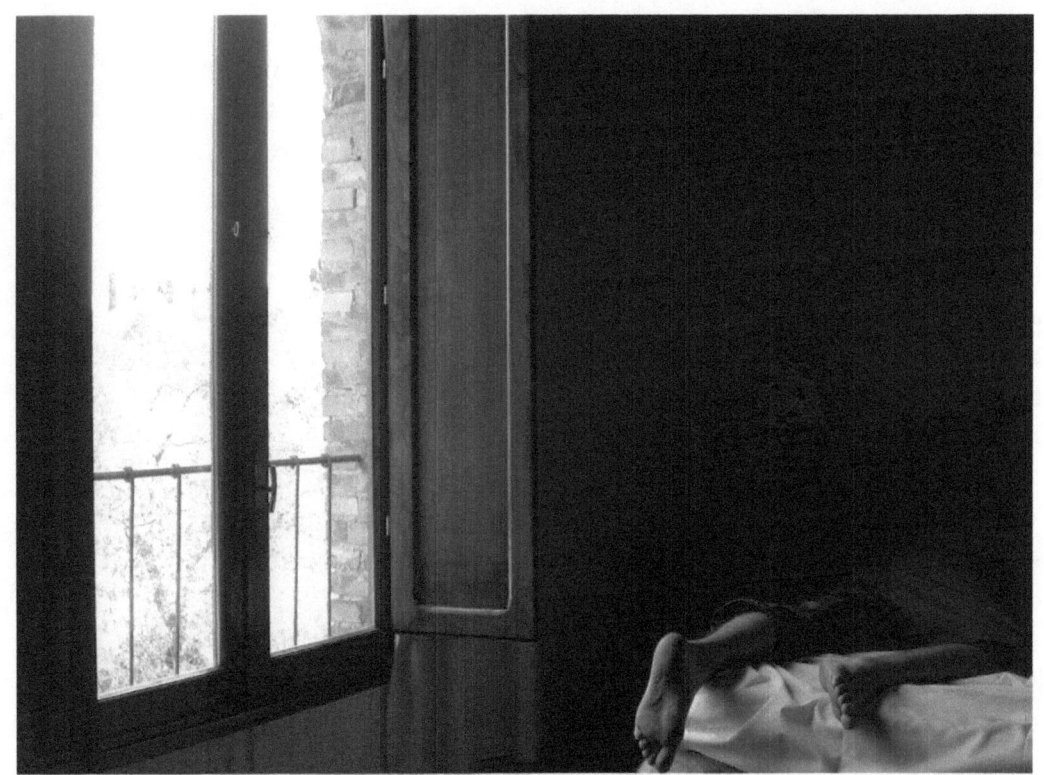

Chapter 7:

I Had This Awesome Dream Last Night!

Synopsis

When we sleep, we surrender ourselves to a parallel universe. We do not control ourselves when we sleep. We submit ourselves to our surroundings, to the people around us, to our environments.

And then we dream. Dreams are an enigmatic area of study even today. No one knows for sure why we dream and what these dreams mean, if anything at all.

We do not know for sure why we get pleasant dreams sometimes and nightmares some other times. There is also no reason (none that we know of) for why we get dreams on some nights and don't on some others. Sleep experts conjecture that we dream all the time—as soon as we go into the sleep mode—but we do not remember most of these dreams when we wake up.

So, why do some dreams leave an impression on our minds, enough for us to remember them when we wake them, and some are forgotten altogether?

There are other problems as well. People do not have the same kind of sleeping habits. Some people sleep fitfully, while others sleep with complete abandon.

Any single person won't sleep in the same manner every night. Our sleep is as varied as it can be, only we do not realize it most of the

time because when we sleep, we are completely in a transcendental stage, an altogether different world.

Why do some people wake up shrieking in the middle of the night, bathed in cold sweat? Why do some people smile when they are sleeping? Why do some people toss restlessly when they are sleeping? Why do some people walk in their sleep?

These are all mysteries that modern science still does not have concrete answers for. We do not know why these things happen. We do not have any rational answers for why these kinds of things happen to one person and do not happen to another.

We shall be taking a closer look at such problems in this chapter.

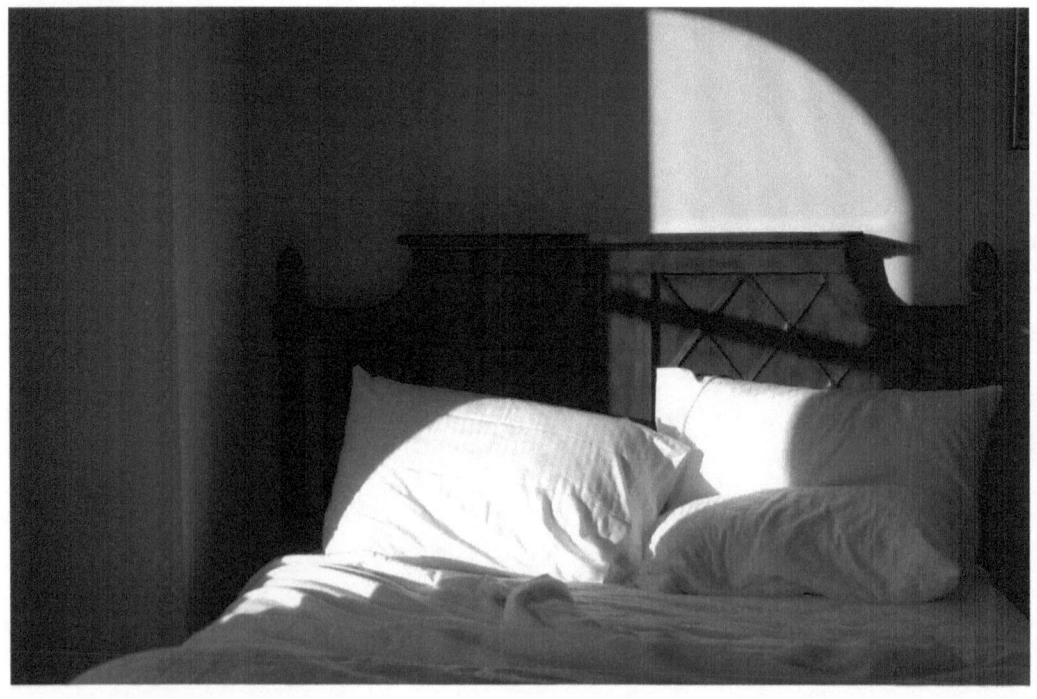

I Had This Awesome Dream Last Night!

Most people spend about 2 hours a night dreaming, although for many of us remembering a dream may be unusual. Why we dream is still the subject of many studies and research projects, however, over the past 30 years research has helped us understand a great deal about dreams and the place of dreaming in our waking and sleeping cycle.

Until recently it was thought that sleep caused all bodily functions to sleep and to rest. Today it is known that far from being a rest time, much of the normal body functions continue as we sleep. This includes our brains, which continue to be active throughout the night.

When we sleep we pass through five stages of sleep, the last one of these stages is called "REM" or Random Eye Movement sleep that is characterized by rapid eye movements and our heart and breath rate rises, our blood pressure rises and this is the stage that we have dreams.

Throughout the night, our sleep cycles through these five stages. The first two are light sleep stages, and the third and fourth stages are typically the sleep we refer to as "deep sleep". The fifth stage is the REM sleep. As the night progresses, the period of REM sleep increases and the period of deep sleep decreases.

People, particularly children who are woken or disturbed during deep sleep will often hallucinate and experience night terrors or nightmares.

Different nerve cells in the brain (known as neurotransmitters) carry the signal to move from stage to stage in the sleep cycles. The messages they carry can be affected by the things we eat and drink, and by such external stimuli as light and noise and for those who smoke, nicotine addiction. These affect the amount of time we spend in REM and it is known that we need the REM sleep for healthy living.

When deprived of REM sleep, laboratory rats died very quickly. People, who are sleep deprived as a form of torture, will also have less REM sleep. REM sleep is essential for optimal memory and brain function. Lack of REM sleep leaves us feeling tired and lethargic throughout the day. It impairs our memory and our judgment and affects our mood. The person who does not have chronic insomnia, will usually require extra "catch up" sleep, after experiencing consecutive days with reduced sleep.

The important factor in ensuring you get enough sleep is to recognize and accept the importance of sleep. Your body relies on sleep to function properly and depriving it of sleep to get things done, will actually have the reverse effect. To achieve the "to do" list effectively and safely, you must sleep. Accept that your physical and mental wellbeing depends on your having the right amount of sleep at night and do your best to set up your life routines to accommodate adequate time to sleep the recommended hours for your age group.

Chapter 8:

There Are Only 24 Hours in a Day

Synopsis

At the end of it all, we need to realize that we only have 24 hours in our day. All our days are the same, at least when we talk about the quantity of time that we have with us per day. But, we may be busier on some days than on others.

We may have an important social function on one day and nothing to do on the other day. Whatever the nature of our day might be, one thing is certain—we just have 24 hours every day to do what we want.

That is the reason we have to become effective time managers. We have to make sure that we plan our routines in such a way that we are able to make the most of it. We have to be able to manage our sleep timings and work timings in such a manner that both get adequate importance.

Upsetting the balance just won't do. Both parts of our life are vitally important to our existence, and we cannot undermine that fact under any circumstances.

There Are Only 24 Hours in a Day

If you are finding yourself tired during the day, yawning during meetings, or overly drowsy when working in a warm room, it's possible you are "sleep deprived". Sleep deprivation is probably one of the most common side effects of our super busy lifestyles. While many people consider that "feeling tired all the time" is a cheap price to pay for being a high achiever, reality is, over time, sleep deprivation will create health problems that will increase over time.

Many people do not realize how little they sleep over the course of a week and it may help to track your own sleeping habits using a sleep diary. In your diary, record when you go to sleep each night and when you wake up the next morning. Document if you need an alarm clock to wake you up and how long it took you approximately to fall asleep. Describe in your diary how you are feeling during the day and especially record the foods you eat and when during the day you feel tired.

Over time, you will observe your own unique cycle to enable you to plan your life choices around that cycle. Plan time in your daily schedule to have a set wake up time and bedtime and if possible create a naptime each afternoon. Prioritize your regulated sleep times and do not compromise on them.

Create routines in your day and include meal times. Increase the amount of fruit and vegetables, good oils and proteins in your diet and reduce the amount of carbohydrates, particularly those that are highly refined white carbohydrates like white bread or rice. Ensure you have time to exercise regularly.

Doctors have described a condition known as "sleep debt". This describes the sleep you do not get during the week compared to what is an average amount of sleep required for your age group. Debt always implies that something must be repaid, and in this context, a lack of sleep must be repaid. Over the course of a year, this may account for two weeks less sleep and the result can be weight gain, impaired vision, raised blood pressure insulin resistance, and cardiac disease.

To enable your body to reestablish a waking sleeping cycle, and to restore normal REM sleep, research has shown that it is important to make up the lost sleep. It is not enough to consider a sleep in on the weekend will repay the debt of a week where you may have slept only a few hours a day.

Research suggests that to reverse the effects of sleep deprivation, you must repay for all the hours or sleep you missed, which effectively means, increase the amount of sleep you have each night for an extended period of time.

You will notice your body starts to form a cycle of waking and sleeping again. You will begin to feel energized and less tired all the time and your health will improve.

Wrapping Up

A healthy sleep is most essential to our wellbeing. We just cannot walk on the wild side too much... we cannot rob our bodies of the sleep that it needs. If we do that too often, our body is naturally going to rebel. Our bodies and minds do not work in tandem most of the time.

Though our mind might tell you that a particular approaching deadline is important and that we need to stay awake to do what we should, our body is not going to understand it. It is going to revolt in its own way if we listen too much to our mind and ignore the needs of our body.

And that is not going to be good for the mind either. When the body revolts, the mind is definitely going to feel the pressure as well. The effects of the body's rebellion will be manifested on the mind in various ways—stress, depression, lack of concentration, lethargy, feeling of extreme tiredness and even phobias and lack of creativity and productivity.

In the world of blatant competition such as what we live in, this kind of loss of skill and talent just won't do. We cannot sit back and let our health take control of us.

Hence, it is important for us to realize that sleep is important. Sleep is not just a waste of time, a time when we do 'nothing'. On the contrary, this is the time when our body is getting charged up. Even as we sleep, various metabolic functions are taking place in our body and they are handling the wear and tear of the body. They are repairing it

with the various mechanisms they have available to them. The body is also working silently, and enhancing itself in various ways.

Also, the mind is working when we are sleeping. It works subconsciously. We create thoughts and ideas as we sleep. A part of our productivity—in fact, the most creative part of our productivity—is generated when we sleep.

In conclusion, sleep isn't something that you should undermine. It isn't something that can be taken lightly. We have to try at all times to schedule our day so that we can work in a healthy sleep pattern in it.

The returns of such an endeavor are immense. We grow in health, and we are able to spend a better and more productive time and effort for whatever we do.

Hopefully, this e-Book has emphasized on the importance of sleep and guided you in ways where you can improve your sleeping patterns.

All the best to you!